Natural

Alkaline Diets, Water & Medicinal Herbs *for*

Herpes

Detoxify, Cleanse and Nourish Blood, Organs and the Entire Body to be Completely Free from Herpes Virus.

Esther Gbemy

Copyright © 2022

Table of Contents

Introduction

Infections with the herpes virus, particularly herpes simplex, are common and afflict 65 to 85% of adults globally. The HSV 1 and HSV 2 herpes viruses are among the two that afflict men. Compared to HSV 2, HSV 1 is far more prevalent.

About 60% of people in the US are affected by the virus. Genital ulcers, skin sores, facial sores, eye sores, and CNS infection are all primarily brought on by this virus.

Unprotected sexual relationship, skin-to-skin contact, kissing an infected person, bodily fluid contact with an infected person, and many more situations can lead to infection.

Increased consumption of iron meals and bodily purification are two benefits of using an alkaline diet. If the necessary foods are not consumed as directed, some herbs are very effective against the herpes virus, but the cure may take a while.

Herpes virus prevention is pretty easy. Some easy strategies to avoid coming into touch with this virus include using condoms, avoiding unprotected intercourse, avoiding numerous partners, and avoiding direct contact with bodily fluids of those who are infected.

In this book, I am going to discuss extensively on the fundamentals of herpes virus, its causes, symptoms, risk factors and as well as the use of alkaline diets that are capable to treat Herpes virus.

Chapter 1

Herpes Virus Fundamentals

Herpes Simplex Virus causes the long-lasting illness known as herpes (HSV). The areas of the body that are harmed by this virus include the vaginal region, the oral region, the skin, and the anal region.

This illness has been around for a very long time and it frequently affects people, creating a variety of illnesses, some of which are deadly and others of which are moderate.

One of the most prevalent herpes simplex virus strains is genital herpes. A sexually transmitted infection that causes genital and anal blisters is the genital herpes virus. Sores that also affect the mouth and face might exist.

HVS 2 is responsible for certain instances of genital herpes that recur. The majority of this virus is transferred by patients who are unaware that they are infected, and most of the time, a patient's symptoms are silent.

Through sexual interaction with an HSV-1 patient, anyone can get this illness. Additionally, if your sex partner has no symptoms at all, you might get the virus from them.

The second form, furthermore, might be brought on by anal-anal or oral-anal contact with a patient. One of the most prevalent herpes virus infection is HSV 2, while HSV 1 infections are less frequent.

In the whole world, genital herpes is one of the most common sexually transmitted illnesses. Herpes simplex virus type 2 (HSV-2) is most commonly responsible for its occurrence, however HSV-1 is also capable of doing so.

When the virus is inoculated onto wet epithelium during close sexual intercourse, genital herpes infections commonly result.

Even while genital herpes infections seldom result in death, they pose a serious threat to public health. Primary acquisition may result in uncomfortable genital ulcers and systemic symptoms including fever and headache.

As the virus becomes latent in the sacral nerve ganglia, infection is regarded as a lifelong condition that can cause repeated genital sores as well as serious psychological discomfort.

HSV transmission during the womb can result in infant mortality or lasting neurological impairment. Additionally, there is proof that HSV infection promotes HIV incidence and sexual transmission.

What are the Major Categories of Herpes Virus?

There are different categories of Herpes virus. These include:

Varicella zoster

1. Shingles.

2. Chicken pox.

Herpes simplex 1 and 2

1. Cold sores.

2. Genital sores.

Epstein-Barr virus

1. Mononucleosis

2. Burkitt's lymphoma.

How Does the Herpes Simplex Virus Occur?

There are different ways in which this virus can be contracted. These include the following:

- Direct touch with the fluid on the genital and anus surfaces.
- Herpes virus can be contracted by close contact with an infected person's bodily fluids.
- Using eyeglasses belonging to an infected individual.
- A sexual partnership involving numerous partners.
- Having an oral sex connection with someone who has mouth sores.

How Herpes Virus is Expressed?

Herpes virus symptoms can appear in one of three ways.

- This happens as a result of viral mutation. Because mistakes in reproducing their RNA genomes are not caught by proofreading, RNA viruses often have an abnormally high rate of mutation. Even in those who are resistant to the virus, certain mutations turn existing viruses into new genetic types that might cause disease.

- Herpes virus transmission from a tiny, isolated human population. For example, AIDS was unnamed and unrecognized for decades until it started to spread globally. Therefore, a previously uncommon human disease was able to spread throughout the world due to technological and social factors like affordable international travel, blood transfusions, sexual immorality, and the abuse of intravenous drugs.

- The transmission of pre-existing virus from other animals. According to scientific estimates, this is how around three-quarters of new human illnesses begin. The term "natural reservoir" refers to an animal that can host and spread a certain virus but is otherwise unaffected by it.

Herpes Virus Infection Dormancy in a Patients Body

The dormancy mechanism is provided by herpes simplex viruses, which get established in sensory neurons in humans.

Most cases of oral herpes are brought on by the type 1 virus, whereas most cases of genital herpes are brought on by the type 2 virus.

The infected cells are ineffective in presenting viral antigens to circulatory lymphocytes because the sensory neurons express comparatively few Major Histocompatibility Complex (MHC) 1 molecules.

The virus and infections of the surrounding epithelial tissues are reactivated by stimuli like fever, mental stress, or menstruation. Blisters around the mouth that is incorrectly referred to as cold sores can appear when the type 1 virus is activated.

Although type 2 viruses can cause vaginal sores, persons who have either type 1 or 2 viruses are frequently asymptomatic.

Sexually transmitted type 2 virus infections offer a major risk to the offspring of infected mothers and can promote the spread of HIV, the virus that causes AIDS.

Symptoms of Herpes Virus

Some signs of this illness that may be seen even if they are occasionally not symptomatic include:

- Awkward vaginal discharge.
- Skin blisters that are red in hue.
- Cold, itchy sores on the lips and mouth.
- Illness.
- Tickling and burning in the vaginal area.
- Anus or rectum inflammation.
- Aches and pains in the afflicted body part.
- Genital sores.
- The development of an ulcer as soon as a blister breaks.
- Muscle pain.

- Problems urinating.

- A rise in temperature.

- Urination that hurts.

- The presence of cervix blisters.

- The lymph nodes expand.

- Itches in the irritated parts.

Chapter 2

Herpes Virus and Central Nervous System

One of the really dangerous HSV infections is encephalitis, and HSV is thought to be the most frequent cause of spontaneous, fatal encephalitis. The HSV encephalitis symptoms in older kids and adults are an indication of the afflicted brain.

Focal encephalitis is the most common of these symptoms, and it is characterized by fever, altered awareness, strange behavior, impaired mentation, and isolated neurological findings.

HSV-1 replicates actively in brain neuronal cells, resulting in herpetic simplex encephalitis (HSE).

Acute HSE caused by HSV-1, which is significant, often affects the temporal and frontal lobes of the brain as well as the insular cortex of the cerebral hemispheres. It results in neuronal cell death by necrosis or apoptosis.

Localized temporal lobe illness is seen in the clinical signs and symptoms. Although there are no pathognomonic symptoms for HSV encephalitis, a rapidly declining level of awareness coupled with a fever and an aberrant CSF profile, in the absence of other reasons, should raise serious concerns about this illness. Since other curable conditions might mimic HSV encephalitis, diagnostic testing should start quickly.

Herpes Virus and its Recurrence

The HSV virus enters a human cell, enters the nucleus, and starts replicating inside the cell. Even while cells may be infected at this point, you most likely won't notice any symptoms.

During the first infection, the virus travels via nerve cells to ganglia, which are nerve-branching locations. The virus will remain inactive and latent there, not multiplying or showing any symptoms that it is even present.

The virus may occasionally abruptly reawaken and begin replicating itself. When this occurs, the virus will return to the skin's surface through the nerve. Blisters develop as a result of the death of many diseased skin cells.

These blisters rupture, resulting in the distinctive ulcers that are known as cold sores or genital herpes.

What Leads to Recurrence?

The herpes virus may reactivate in response to specific circumstances. Even if your immune system is in good shape, this is referred to as a recurrence.

Several recognized triggers, such as the following, have been shown to induce recurrence:

- ✓ Weakness (fatigue).
- ✓ Being exposed to extreme heat, cold, or UV radiation (such as that from the sun).
- ✓ Physical strain brought on by an accident, disease, or infection.
- ✓ Prolonged emotional tension or worry that lasts longer than a week.
- ✓ Hormonal changes, such those that occur during menstruation.

Herpes Virus Danger Signs

If you already have HSV-1 or HSV-2, there are a number of health conditions that can make it more likely that your HSV infection will be more severe or stay longer. However, none of these risk factors increase your likelihood of contracting the illness. As follows:

Use of immunosuppressive drugs

If you use immunosuppressive drugs like steroids or chemotherapy, your HSV-1 or HSV-2 infection might get worse or reactivate.

Once you stop taking the drug and your immune system starts functioning normally, this should no longer be the case.

Immunosuppression

You run a higher chance of developing a more serious or long-lasting HSV infection as well as more frequent reactivations if your immune system is compromised for any reason.

An autoimmune disorder, HIV, immunoglobulin A (IgA) disease, a sickness like bone marrow malignancy, chemotherapy, or organ transplantation are a few conditions that might weaken your immune system.

Human Immunodeficiency Virus (HIV)

HIV infection in particular results in lowered viral immunity, and herpes virus infections might become more severe if you have HIV.

Sharing objects

Sharing objects like cups, toothbrushes, and even towels that have previously been exposed to the virus can spread the HSV-1 virus. It is especially dangerous to use someone else's lipstick, lip gloss, or lip balm since they are naturally wet and the virus can readily attach to them.

Long-term skin-to-skin contact

The sores on the face, head, and neck are a hallmark of the HSV-1 infection known as Herpes gladiatorum. Wrestlers are more frequently reported to have this particular herpes virus.

IgA Deficiency

Although any immune disorder may put you at risk for recurring sores or a more severe case of HSV infection, IgA deficiency is the immunological disorder that is most frequently linked to HSV.

IgA is an immunological protein that primarily guards against infections of the mucous membranes, or the thin skin parts that are covered in a fluid-like mucus, including the mouth and vagina.

Unprotected sex

Sexual activity, especially oral sex, is the main way that HSV-2 is passed from one person to another. Although it is less often, HSV-1 may also be spread during intercourse. Multiple sexual partners and unprotected intercourse with potential infected partners increase your risk.

Kissing

One of the most typical methods of transmitting HSV-1 is by kissing or other mouth-to-mouth contact.

The Relationship between the Immune System and Herpes Virus

Your body's defense against bacteria, fungi, poisons, and viral illnesses is the immune system. It fights these many foreign things that may infect you or hurt you by involving a variety of organs, cells, proteins, and tissues.

Your immune system targets and regulates everything you consume or touch, and it does this continuously.

Viruses often infect cells when they enter your body. Your immune system responds by identifying, binding to, and destroying the infected cells through the action of your T cells.

Things are little more difficult when you have a herpes infection, though. This is because herpesviruses hinder certain cells from realizing they are infected when they infect them.

They may conceal and, in a sense, sleep this way. The virus can therefore evade your immune system's identification.

The virus can remain in your system for such a long time in this way. Although it could be in your body, it seldom causes any problems.

Things don't start until it transitions from its latency phase, or that slumber, to its activation phase. For instance, your cold sore appears, you become infectious, and your immune system tries to eradicate the virus when you are worried, exhausted, or weak.

There is proof, for instance, that the cytomegalovirus (CMV), one kind of herpes, may compromise your immune system.

Although CMV is one of the most prevalent types of herpesvirus, it does not produce the typical signs and symptoms of that illness. Instead, it mostly affects infants, who may experience developmental delays as well as vision and hearing issues.

Latent CMV may make your body less able to fight off other illnesses since it is just too busy battling this virus, claims one research.

But there's an issue with this. According to research, between 50 and 90 percent of us carry the virus latently throughout our lifetime.

This means that its real effects are much more challenging to determine, as everyone's immune system is fighting the virus to a degree.

Chapter 3

What are Alkaline Diets?

Within a relatively small range, the pH is tightly regulated in all biological fluids and tissues.

Additionally, each kind of cell, tissue, and organ, such as the stomach, muscles, and blood, has a certain ideal pH level. The act of maintaining pH within a specific range is known as acid-alkaline balance or acid-alkaline homeostasis.

Foods that are alkaline have a tonic impact on the body. Alkaline foods balance blood acidity, which acts as a breath of fresh air for the body, regenerating and repairing damaged cells. Acid-rich diets speed up the breakdown of bodily cells, resulting in acid bombs that circulate in the circulation and wreck havoc on the body.

Alkaline diets are those that exclude all meals that contain acids completely. They are also known as "electric meals" because they support the body's innate ability to repair itself. They are not altered, hybridized, or exposed to radiation; they are just present in nature.

Alkaline meals help the body absorb more iron, copper, and other vital vitamins and minerals that strengthen the immune system.

They are meals that raise the alkalinity of your blood, which protects you against illnesses and infections as many pathogens prefer an acidic environment to grow.

Finding foods that have an alkalizing impact on the body can aid in preserving ideal blood pH levels.

The term "alkaline diet" refers to a way of eating that focuses on giving the body the nutrition and sustenance it needs to stay healthy, energetic, and vibrant.

People benefit from an improved acid-alkaline balance in their bodies by having better immunity, more energy, and less pain.

Alkaline diets improved skeletal health by reducing osteoporosis and arthritis pain, improved digestion and the reduction of gastrointestinal pain from acid reflux, ulcers, and bowel issues, improved nutrient uptake, and improved detoxification by restoring the body's pH balance.

When the blood maintains a "normal or slightly alkaline pH," any chronic sickness in humans can be cured.

What Advantages does an Alkaline Diet have?

Alkaline diets have the following advantages:

- Treats and prevents the herpes simplex virus

- Does not contain cholesterol.

- It is alcohol-free.

- Has a very low fat content that protects against heart disease and other cardiac problems.

- Prevents cancer and treats it.

- Prevents stroke and treats it.

- Lowers blood pressure and avoids it.

- Has very little saturated fat, which helps to prevent serious heart diseases.

- It is free of refined sugar.

- Treats and prevents diabetes.

- Make the majority of those who follow the program experience weight loss.

What Diets Are Acidic?

Acidic foods are those with a high acid content and are frequently bad for human health. Increased levels of body acid make it simple for infectious illnesses to spread, flourish, and develop. Since they could reduce the efficacy of the meals and herbal items. I'll mention the kinds of items that are not allowed in a fully alkaline diet in the chapter above. Acidic foods include those that are off-limits.

Body pH Levels

The pH scale determines whether a food item is acidic or alkaline.

The pH scale goes from 0 to 14, with 7 being regarded neutral, 7 being considered acidic, and 7 being considered alkaline.

An essential idea in pH is that a pH value over 7 is 10 times more alkaline and a pH value below 7 is 10 times more acidic than the next higher number. A pH of 4 is 10 times more acidic than a pH of 5, and a pH of 6 is 100 times more acidic.

As a result, even minor pH changes can have a big influence on health.

Relationship between an Alkaline Diet and The Herpes Virus

Diets high in alkalinity are crucial for the treatment of the herpes virus. Alkaline diets aid in cleansing the body down to the cellular level and aid the body in removing any mucus-forming substances. When trying to treat the herpes virus, these diets shouldn't be ignored.

However, an alkaline diet alone cannot treat these illnesses; however, when fasting and the use of detoxifying herbs are combined, a cure for these infections is certain.

Additionally, the oxygen content that these viruses require to develop, reproduce, and propagate will be eliminated. As a result, the body is given the ingredients it needs to combat sickness.

What Foods Are Excluded From An Alkaline Diet?

Many foods that are not naturally alkaline are excluded from a comprehensive alkaline diet regimen. The majority of the things you eat are quite acidic, which slows down the body's ability to recover and mend itself. Alkaline diets ban the following foods:

- Poultry products.
- Alcoholic beverages.
- Soy and soy-based goods.
- Corn.
- Seafood and fish.
- Flavors and colors.
- Meat of many varieties.
- Eggs.
- Processed food
- Fruits in tins.
- Fruits without seeds.
- Foods containing yeast or other ingredients, such baking powder.
- Wheat.

- Quick meals.

- Vegetables made with genetically modified organisms.

- Dairy goods.

- Sugar.

- Supplemented vitamins and minerals in food

- Garlic.

- Fruits made from genetically modified organisms.

Balance Between Acid And Alkalinity

Within a certain range, the pH level is managed in biological fluids and tissues. Additionally, each type of cell, tissue, and organ, such as the stomach, muscles, and blood, has a specific ideal pH level. Arterial blood typically has a pH between 7.35 and 7.45.

Acid-alkaline balance or acid-alkaline homeostasis refers to the act of maintaining pH within a specific range.

The human body has a number of natural buffer systems that contribute to homeostasis, which is preserved through the metabolic and respiratory systems of the kidneys, lungs, and other tissues.

The hydrogen ions are bound by the buffering substances, which lessens the possibility of pH fluctuations. According to reports, acidification of bio-fluids in the human body might have a variety of negative consequences.

Reasons why Diets are Alkaline

Low in Sugar

Sugar, whether it be glucose, fructose, or dextrose, is sugar, and all sugar regardless of its form produces significant amounts of acid in the body.

Fresh Foods

Fresh foods tend to be more alkali-forming since all of their nutrients are present. They can occasionally, but not always, be processed to become acidic. This is especially true for meals that include oils, which turn hazardous when exposed to heat, light, and air.

Mineral Content

The main reason why alkaline foods are alkaline is because they are high in alkaline minerals. Calcium, magnesium, potassium, sodium bicarbonate, manganese, and iron are the minerals with the highest alkalinity.

Vegetables

Since almost all vegetables range from moderate to extremely alkaline-forming, they can be consumed in large quantities.

High Water Content

Foods with high water content tend to have a higher alkali forming potential.

Foods with a green color that contain chlorophyll are also very alkaline.

Can you eat an Alkaline Diet if your Stomach is Acidic?

In order to digest the food consumed and get it ready for nutrient extraction in the large intestine, the stomach creates hydrochloric acid on demand. As demonstrated by in vitro studies, the stomach acid just prepares the meal for the next stage of digestion, during which nutrients such as alkaline minerals, antioxidants, and vitamins are drawn out and distributed throughout the body.

In comparison to alkaline meals like celery, spinach, cucumbers, kale, watercress, lettuce, and carrots, the stomach must create more hydrochloric acid to digest acidic foods like red wine, sweets, cakes, ice cream, chocolate, pizza, chips, fast food, and so on.

The body might experience extreme stress as a result of the ongoing overproduction of hydrochloric acid and the subsequent neutralization procedure. Heartburn and acid reflux symptoms may appear as a result, and they may quickly worsen.

The alkaline diet encourages consuming large amounts of fruits, vegetables, and nutritious plant foods while limiting processed junk food.

The assertions regarding the mechanism underlying the diet, however, are not supported by evolutionary data, human physiology, or any reputable human studies. In fact, acids, such as amino acids, fatty acids, and DNA, are among the most significant components of life.

The alkaline diet is beneficial because it emphasizes eating whole, unprocessed foods.

How to Eliminate Anything that Cause Disease and Avoid Symptoms

The majority of ill disorders have formed as a result of self-generated poisons produced by undigested meals, thus we must first learn how to "eliminate the cause."

This only implies that we must cease consuming "acid-forming meals," which cause our body tissue to become acidic and so suffocate our body cells' ability to absorb oxygen.

Diets that produce acid are the main underlying factor in the majority of illnesses. In order to cure the cause and symptoms, we must first understand the fundamentals of how to do it.

The ability of your immune system to guard and fight itself against all causes and circumstances of disease is crippled as a result of low quality, poisonous body cells; learning how to address these causes can help you prevent this. Learn how to consume alkaline foods, stop

35

eating acid-forming meals, and lead a toxic-free existence.

Chapter 4

Lists of Some Alkaline Diets

These alkaline diets are classified into a number of categories such as: Fruits, herbs, vegetables, grains, sweeteners, herbal teas, seasonings, and spices are among these categories.

Lists of some Alkaline Diets		
Spices & Seasoning	**Fruits**	**Vegetable**
Pure Sea Salt, Dill, Achiote, Habanero, Savory, Basil, Thyme, Bay Leaf Cayenne Cloves,	Prickly Pear, Cherries, Orange, Soft Jelly Coconuts, Papayas, Melons, Figs, Grapes, Sour sups, Prunes, Bananas, Dates,	Dulse, Garbanzo Beans, Arame, Wild, Arugula, Cherry and Plum Tomato, Cucumber, Wakame, Lettuce except for the Iceberg, Nori, Avocado, Izote flower and leaf, Kale, Mushrooms except for Shitake,

Onion Powder, Sweet Basil, Oregano, Powdered Granulated Seaweed and Tarragon. Sage.

Cantaloupe, Apples, Pears, Limes, Currants, Peaches, Plums, Mango, Berries, Rasins.

Bell Pepper, Chayote, Zucchini, Nopales, Olives, Dandelion Greens, Amaranth, Watercress, Tomatillo, Turnip Greens, Onions, Squash, Okra, Hijiki, Purslane, Verdolaga.

Grains

Wild Rice, Spelt, Fonio, Tef, Kamut, Amaranth, Quinoa & Rye.

Herbs

Dill, Onion powder, Basil, Cayenne, Pure sea salt & Oregano

Herbs Tea

Ginger, Burdock, Chamomile, Fennel, Red Raspberry, Elderberry & Tila.

Sweeteners

Date Sugar, Agave Syrup from cactus (100% Pure).

Essential Method Employed for the Treatment of Herpes Virus

There are some essential methods you can follow in order to fight against herpes virus. These methods include:

- Detoxification.
- The use of therapeutic herbs.

After the last therapy for these viruses, basic alkaline diets must be consumed. As you are not encouraged to resume eating the meals you did before to the start of this therapy, doing so will enable the treatment to be perfected.

In this instance, the next chapters will detail specific meals that are crucial for you once the therapy is over.

Alkaline Detoxification Herbs for Herpes Virus

He uses detoxification as his initial strategy for treating the herpes virus. The colon is the main organ that alkaline herbs purify, but because the detoxification process is completely holistic, it also cleanses the liver, gall bladder, kidneys, and lymph glands.

To rid the body of any infection, the intracellular level of the body must be cleaned.

By enabling the body to reorganize itself after consuming enough sea moss plant, alkaline herbs aid in stimulating the body.

Two Weeks Fasting Detoxification for Herpes Virus

Fasting is a crucial component that might aid in the body's detoxification. When you fast, your body goes through a detoxification and cleaning process. You must make sufficient sacrifices, such as the one you are going to make, in order to overcome this sickness.

Depending on how seriously you utilize the procedures since the virus is difficult to get rid of from the body, you may be able to detox from it. They remain there after attacking the immunological and nervous systems. As a result, your body must escort them out while also waking them up through fasting and cleansing.

These herbs include:

- Nopal plant

- Burdock root.

- Stinging nettle root.

- Elderberry.

- Linden leaf.

- Sea moss plant.

Make careful to give this plant a good rinse with running water after collecting them. You may use direct sunshine to dry them.

Making the Herbs Ready
- Make sure the plants are completely dried off and store them in a dry, sterile container.
- Process them into a powder.
- Combine two cups of alkaline or Spring water with one tablespoon of each of the aforementioned plants.
- Put it near a heat source and wait for it to boil.

- The water should be brought to a boil within three minutes, or as soon as you see that plant extracts are beginning to emerge and the color of the water has changed.

- Although herbs are best consumed when hot since the bitterness will be decreased, remove it from the heat source and let it cool for a few minutes before eating. For two weeks, this should be taken in the morning and right before bed.

- You can also eat a wide variety of other fruits and vegetables throughout this procedure, such as watermelon, berries, mushrooms, zucchini, cactus plants, and leafy greens. Water and tamarind juice are further options.

- Even though they are on the food lists, you are not needed to consume any solid meals during this two weeks of detoxification. Nuts, seeds, and grains are not acceptable foods. You can eat them when the healing procedure is complete.

What Advantages Do Alkaline Detoxifying Herbs Offer?

The herbs mentioned above perform the following functions for the body:

- Rejuvenate the body.

- Eliminate toxins from the body's waste.

- The body's cells multiply.

- Provide the body with irons, which are crucial for the herpes virus's healing.

- Promotes and cleans the blood.

How Long Does It Take To Heal From The Herpes Virus?

The amount of days it will take to be treated depends on the sufferer's weight and general health. Each person's recovery period is unique since each person has a unique health situation.

How long it takes a patient to fully recover from this illness will depend on the state of their pancreas, liver, intestines, and other vital organs.

Practice fasting more; make a strategy and follow through. Fasting increases the speed at which you heal. If you are feeling extremely weak while fasting, you can eat dates.

The Alkaline Therapeutic Herbs for Herpes Virus

Following the completion of the detoxification procedure, you will begin using medicinal herbs that are highly iron-rich.

There are around eleven (11) different kinds of alkaline herbs used to cure herpes. All plants are a great source of iron and potassium phosphate. Here is a list of these herbs:

- Sarsil berry.
- Sarsasparilla.
- Guaco.
- Conconsa.
- Purslane.
- Kale.
- Dandelion.

- The Lams Quarters.

- Burdock.

- Yellow dock.

- Blue vervain.

Making the Herbs Ready

- Make sure the plants are completely dried off and store them in a dry, sterile container.

- Powder the herbs by grinding them.

- Four glasses of Spring water should be added along with one teaspoon of each of the aforementioned plants.

- Put it near a heat source and wait for it to boil.

- The water should be brought to a boil within three minutes, or as soon as you see the release of plant extracts and a change in the color of the water.

- •

- Though herbs are best consumed when hot since the bitterness will be minimized, remove it from the heat source and let it cool for a few minutes before consuming.

- Until you feel better, take these herbs twice day with a glass cup.

How Well Do These Herbs Work For Treating Herpes?

Blue Vervain

Iron is abundant in this plant.

Berry Sarsil

Because it is a berry from the Sarsaparilla plant, this plant contains iron. This plant helps in treating herpes.

Guaco Plant

This plant has a high iron content, which boosts immunity, and potassium phosphate, which makes it effective against the herpes virus.

Sarsaparilla

Herpes simplex and genital herpes are treated with this plant because it has the greatest iron content.

Sarsaparilla may have therapeutic effects on syphilis, herpes, rheumatic illnesses, passive general dropsy, and gonorrheal rheumatism, according to research.

Triterpenes, sarsaparilloside, parillin, smitilbin, and phenolic compounds are the active components of this plant that make it beneficial against herpes.

Conconsa

This plant is native to Africa. It is embedded with the largest amount of potassium phosphate, which inhibits the herpes virus.

Purslane

Iron content is abundant in purslane. According to herbalists, this plant is efficient in treating herpes simplex.

Kale plant

Iron antioxidants are abundant in this plant. Additionally, it has higher lysine, which is a crucial amino acid ratio for inhibiting the herpes virus. Lysine is an amino acid that aids in preventing the body's herpes virus cells from proliferating.

Yellow Dock

Iron is abundant in this plant.

Lams Quarters

Iron is abundant in this plant.

Burdock Plant

Iron is abundant in this plant.

Effectiveness of Dandelion Root in the Treatment of Herpes

Iron and potassium are abundant in this plant. It is one of the most well-known herbs that is crucial for the recovery from many ailments. Skin wounds have been treated using it in the past. Along with aiding in the removal of toxins from the body, this plant is a crucial component in the treatment of liver disorders.

Dandelion also aids in the elimination of kidney and bladder stones. It contributes to decreasing high blood pressure.

This plant has been widely utilized in alternative medicine to cure a variety of conditions in many people, including hypoglycemia, breast cancer, herpes, HIV/AIDS, hypertension, and herpes.

Laxative, stomachic, alterative, cholagogue, diuretic, choleretic, anti-inflammatory, antioxidant, anti-carcinogenic, analgesic, anti-hyperglycemic, anti-coagulatory, and prebiotic are some of the qualities this plant possesses.

The active ingredients present in this plant are:

Carotenoids, Taraxsterol, Asparagine, Choline, Tannins, Sterols, Araxacin, Triterpenes and Taraxol.

Dandelion's Effectiveness in Treating Herpes: Scientific Evidence

The Jiangxi Medical College conducted research. On the type 1 herpes simplex virus, they tested a number of therapeutic plants. Dandelion has been identified as one of the herbs that are beneficial against herpes after several screenings.

Needed Information and Advice for Absolute Cure of Herpes Virus

Consume meals that are on the list of alkaline foods once you've finished the entire process, including the fast and the intake of therapeutic herbs.

Fruits, smoothies, and vegetables should be the only things you eat following treatment; solid meals should not be consumed in large quantities or should only be a small portion of your diet.

You must eliminate from your diet any items that naturally produce acids. Verify the list of banned foods from the chapter before.

Take good care of your health and happiness. To reach your goal, emotional equilibrium is necessary.

Do your best to avoid skipping the fast or forgetting to take your herbs.

Chapter 5

Alkaline Diets for Herpes Virus

There are a variety of diets that can help you prevents and treats herpes virus. Diets may be made from any of alkaline food lists. Because his meals are alkaline and capable of cleansing and eliminating viruses from the body, they should not be over-emphasized.

Number 1. Alkaline Ingredients

1.	1 cupful of almond milk	5.	6 tbsp. of Agave Nectar
2.	2 cupsful of Spelt flour	6.	6 Strawberries sliced into sizes.
3.	1 tsp. of Vanilla extract.	7.	6 tbsp. of water.
4.	1 tsp. of sea moss.		

How to make it

- Fill a container halfway with the Spelt flour, Seams, and Strawberry bits.

- Mix together the Vanilla Extract, Agave Nectar, water, and Almond Milk.

- Combine all of the ingredients in a mixing bowl.

- Simmer in a Waffle Maker

- Allow to cool after removing from the heat.

- Serve it.

Number 2. Alkaline Ingredients

1.	4 tbsp. of Almond milk	6.	2 tbsp. of freshly squeezed Lime juice.
2.	4 sprints of Cilantro	7.	1 tsp. of Sea salt.
3.	3 tbsp. of Maple syrup.	8.	1/2 cupful of Olive oil.
4.	2 packets of Spelt penne.	9.	1 cupful of Sun-dried Tomatoes.
5.	2 Avocados cut in sizes.	10.	1cupful of sliced Onions.

How to make it

- Cook the pasta according to the package directions. This is stated in the product's booklet.

- In a large mixing basin, combine all of the ingredients.

- Combine all ingredients in a blender and blend until they are smoothly blended, then serve.

Number 3. Alkaline Ingredients

1.	3 cups of Springwater.	6.	1 tsp. Thyme.
2.	2 tbsp. of Olive oil.	7.	½ red Pepper, chopped.
3.	2 tsp. of Oregano.	8.	½ tsp. of Sea salt.
4.	A pinch of African red pepper.	9.	½ yellow Onion chopped.
5.	1 cup of Wild rice.	10.	½ cup of chopped Mushrooms,

How to make it

- Cook wild rice until it reaches the half-cooked stage (partially done).

- Heat up the olive oil in a cooking saucepan.

- Sauté the carrots and mushrooms for around 2 minutes.
- Stir in the thyme, oregano, sea salt, and red pepper.
- Combine the ingredients in a pot with the prepared rice and simmer for 15 minutes, or until the rice is done.
- Serve it.

Number 4.   Alkaline Ingredients

1.	30 oz. of Mushrooms.	7.	1 bunch of torn Romaine Lettuce.
2.	4 chopped red Onion.	8.	1 bunch of torn fresh Spinach.
3.	2 tsp. of Dill.	9.	1 tsp. of Sea salt
4.	2 red chopped bell pepper.	10.	1 bunch of torn red leaf Lettuce.
5.	2 tsp. of Basil.	11.	½ cup fresh Lime juice.
6.	2 cups of Olive oil.		

How to make it

- Under running water, wash the mushrooms and vegetables to remove any remaining dirt.

- After that, cut them into slices and place them in a dish.

- Toss the Mushroom with the olive oil, lime juice, dill, onion, bell pepper, salt, and basil.

- Refrigerate for 20-30 minutes after mixing the ingredients.

- Serve and have nice fun with it.

Number 5. Alkaline Ingredients

1.	1 cupful of Almond milk.	5.	1 cupful of Sea Moss.
2.	1 cupful of Blueberries.	6.	1 tsp. of Sea Salt.
3.	1 cupful of Kamut flour.	7.	1/2 tsp. of Baking powder.
4.	1 cupful of Spelt flour.	8.	3 tbsp. of Maple syrup.

How to make it

- To begin, preheat the oven to 200 degrees Fahrenheit.
- In a muffin pan, arrange your baking cups.
- Combine the flour, sugar, salt, baking powder, and sea moss in a mixing bowl.
- Mix in the Almond Milk until everything is properly combined. Blueberries are rolled on top.
- Fill the Baking Cups with them.
- Bake for 30–35 minutes, or until done, in a preheated oven.
- Allow to cool after removing from heat.
- Have fun alone.

Number 6.   Alkaline Ingredients

1.	4 tbsp. of Raisins.	4.	2 cupful of Kamut Four.
2.	2 tsp. of Seams powder.	5.	1½ cupful of Almond Milk
3.	2 tsp. of Vanilla extract.	6.	1 cupful of maple crystals.

How to make it

- In a jar, combine the Kamut flour and sea moss powder.

- Combine the raisins, vanilla essence, and maple crystals in a mixing bowl.

- Place the almond milk in a separate basin.

- Combine the two instructions above in the Almond milk container and thoroughly mix.

- Transfer the mixture to a hot pan and cook evenly on both sides.

- Turn off the heat and serve it.

Number 7.   Alkaline Ingredients

1.	4 tsp. of Almond butter.	5.	2 tsp. of cinnamon.
2.	3-4 cupsful of water.	6.	1 tsp. of Sea moss
3.	3 tsp. of Vanilla extract.	7.	1 cupful of maple syrup.
4.	3 cupsful of Almond milk.		

How to make it

- Boil the sea moss in a saucepan.

- Collect and thoroughly combine the cooked sea moss.

- In a blender, combine the remaining ingredients with the pureed Sea moss.

- Blend until the mixture is completely smooth.

- Serve it and take pleasure in it alone.

Number 8.   Alkaline Ingredients

1.	6 cups of sliced Mushrooms.	5.	2 tsp. of Chili powder.
2.	3 tsp. of Onion powder.	6.	2 cups of sliced Onions.
3.	3 tsp. of Sea salt.	7.	2 tbsp. of Oregano.
4.	3 tbsp. of Tomato sauce.	8.	1 tsp. of ground Thyme.

How to make it

- With the use of a saucepan, heat your olive oil.

- Sauté the onion until it begins to color slightly.

- Sauté for a few minutes with the Mushroom.

- Season with salt, pepper, and cayenne pepper.

- Fill a corn shell halfway with the mixture.

- After that, cook till golden brown.

Number 9.   Alkaline Ingredients

1.	15 chopped Cherry Tomatoes.	5.	2 small red and green peppers.
2.	5 tbsp. of Olive oil.	6.	2 cups of chopped Broccoli.
3.	4 sliced Zucchini.	7.	1 sliced small yellow Onion.
4.	2 packs of chopped Oyster Mushrooms.		

How to make it

- In a saucepan, heat your olive oil.

- Stir in the Tomatoes and Onions.

- Season with spices and cook for about 2-3 minutes, stirring occasionally.

- 3 minutes after adding the mushrooms, stir fried them.

- Add bell peppers, zucchini, and broccoli to the pan and cook for another 2-3 minutes.

Number 10.   Alkaline Ingredients

1.	A pinch of Thyme.	6.	1 green Onion.
2.	1 tbsp. of Springwater.	7.	1 pinch of Cumin, Ground
3.	½ tsp. of Maple syrup.	8.	Quarter tsp. of Sweet basil
4.	A pinch of Sea salt.	9	A quarter cup of Fresh Lime juice
5.	2 tbsp. of Almond butter.		

How to make it

- Fill a bottle with spring water and close it.

- Combine all of the ingredients in a bottle and fill with water.

- Enjoy the concoction after shaking it.

1.	16 oz. of sliced Mushrooms.	7.	1 cup of Quinoa
2.	8 oz. of Kamut pasta.	8.	1 bunch of washed and heated Spinach.
3.	4 bunch Kale.	9.	1 small chopped Bell Pepper, red and green.
4.	Three tbsp. of Olive oil	10.	1 Clove.
5.	2 large peeled and chopped Chayote squash.	11.	1 bunch of washed and heated Spinach.
6.	2 sliced Onion.	12	Get Spring Water

How to make it

- Using a saucepan, warm up your oil.

- For 10 minutes, sauté the onions, bell peppers, and mushrooms in the oil, stirring occasionally.

- Fill a cooking saucepan halfway with spring water and add the ingredients listed above.

- Chayote squash should be added at this point.

- Stir in the quinoa, marjoram, oregano, clove, cumin, rosemary, thyme, and red pepper, as well as the remaining ingredients.

- Allow 30 minutes to cook.

- Cook for 10 minutes with Kamut Pasta added.

- Include Spinach and stir them together.

- Serve and take pleasure in the moment.

Number 12.   Alkaline Ingredients

1.	1 cupful of Almond milk.	4.	¼ cupful of Agave nectar.
2.	½ tsp. of Sea moss	5.	¼ cupful of cold water
3.	¼ cupful of fresh Papaya.		

How to make it

- In a blender, combine the water and sea moss.

- Until smooth, blend fully.

- In a blender, combine the remaining recipes.

- Blend until the mixture is completely smooth.

- Instantly take it.

Number 13. Alkaline Ingredients

1.	8 chopped Cherry Tomatoes.	5.	1 pack of chopped Oyster Mushrooms
2.	3 tbsp. of pure Olive oil	6.	1 cupsful of chopped Broccoli
3.	2 chopped Zucchini	7.	1 chopped red and green Pepper.
4.	½ chopped yellow Onion		

How to make it

- In a frying pan, pour the olive oil.

- Stir in the tomatoes and onions. Allow it to cook for a few minutes.

- Sauté for another 5 minutes with the mushrooms.

- Add the bell peppers, broccoli, and zucchini and sauté for another 4 minutes.

- Have fun alone.

Number 14. Alkaline Ingredients

1.	3 bunches of Kale.	7.	1 large Clove.
2.	2 large peeled and sliced Chayote squash.	8.	1 cupful of chopped Oyster Mushrooms.
3.	2 tbsp. of Olive oil.	9.	1 tie of rinsed Spinach, and steamed.
4.	2 slices of Onions.	10.	1 red and green chopped Bell Pepper.
5.	1 cupful of Quinoa.	11.	½ cupful of Kamut Spiral Pasta.
6.	1 tie of rinsed Spinach, and steamed.	12	½ tsp. of mixed spices of your choice.

How to make it

- Heat the olive oil in a pot.

- Mushrooms, bell peppers, and onions should be stir-fried softly for 12 minutes in the oil.

- Fill a soup pot halfway with spring water and add all of the above.

- Chayote Squash should be added at this point.

- Spices should be added now.

- Allow 30-40 minutes for cooking.

- Cook for another 10 minutes with the Kamut Pasta.

- Stir in the Spinach well.

- Serve it.

Number 15.   Alkaline Ingredients

1.	2 tbsp. of agave nectar.	4.	1/2 tsp. of vanilla extract.
2.	1 cup of almond milk.	5.	2 tbsp. of agave nectar.
3.	1 cup of water.		

How to make it

- A cooking pot is used to bring water to a boil.

- Remove the pan from the heat source as soon as it begins to boil.

- Stir in the rye cream until it thickens.

- Combine the remaining ingredients in a large mixing bowl and thoroughly mix them together.

Number 16.   Alkaline Ingredients

1.	2 green and quarter red Bell Pepper	6.	One tsp. of ground Cumin
2.	2 slices of crushed Kamut.	7.	1 lb. of brown button Mushroom
3.	2 tbsp. of Olive oil	8.	1/2 tsp. of Dill.
4.	1/4 tsp. of Sea salt.	9	1/2 cupful of Quinoa.
5.	1/2 cupful of Quinoa.		

How to make it

- To begin, preheat your oven to around 270 degrees Celsius.

- Heat the bell peppers in a saucepan. after that, hollow out

- Pour the water into a saucepan and fill it to three-quarters full.

- Toss in the quinoa grain.

- Cook until all of the water has been absorbed.

- In a skillet, heat the olive oil and sauté the mushrooms and red bell peppers.

- In the olive oil, combine the cumin, bell peppers, and spices.

- Mix the Quinoa, Mushrooms, and Bell Pepper with the remaining ingredients in a large mixing bowl.

- Using your preheated oven, bake the mixture for approximately 12 minutes.

- Allow to cool for a few minutes after removing from the oven.

Number 17.   Alkaline Ingredients

1.	½ cupful of Kamut puff.	4.	1½ tbsp. of Raisins.
2.	½ cupful of hot Almond milk	5.	1½ tbsp. of sliced Dates
3.	1½ tbsp. of Agave nectar.	6.	1½ tbsp. of sliced Almonds.

How to make it

- With the exception of the almond milk, combine all of the ingredients in a mixing bowl and mix well.
- Include Almond milk and drink.

Number 18.   Alkaline Ingredients

1.	1 cupful of Maple crystals.	4.	½ tsp. of Vanilla extract.
2.	1 tsp. of Cinnamon.	5.	4 cupsful of Almond milk.
3.	1 cupful of Kamut flour.	6.	2 cupful of Water.

How to make it

- A cooking pot is used to bring water to a boil.
- Remove from heat after it has reached a boil.
- Mix in the Kamut cream until it thickens up.
- Stir in the rest of the ingredients.
- Serve it.

Number 19. Alkaline Ingredients

1. 6 bunch of Mustard and Turnips greens.
2. 4 cups of sliced Onions.
3. 4 tbsp. of Sea salt.
4. 2 tbsp. of Olive oil.
5. 2 tsp. of Chili powder.

How to make it

- With the use of a saucepan, heat your olive oil.
- Sauté the onion.
- Cook for 10 minutes with the Green Vegetables added.
- Chili powder and salt should be added at this point.
- Remove from the heat after stirring.
- Serve and have a palatable fun.

References

Bruno G. Acid-Alkaline Balance and health: An examination of the data. Supplement Science, 2013, 34-39.

Bradshaw, M. J., and Venkatesan, A. (2016). Herpes simplex virus-1 encephalitis in adults: pathophysiology, diagnosis, and management. *Neurotherapeutics* 13, 493–508. doi: 10.1007/s13311-016-0433-7.

Gnann, J. W., and Whitley, R. J. (2017). Herpes simplex encephalitis: an update. *Curr. Infect. Dis. Rep.* 19:13. doi: 10.1007/s11908-017-0568-7.

Jelang Jelku D Sangma, Jessie Suneetha W and B Anila Kumari. Concepts of acid alkaline diet. Pharma Innovation Journal 2019; 8(4): 932-935.

Koufman JA, Johnston N. Potential benefits of pH 8.8 alkaline drinking water as an adjunct in the treatment of reflux disease. Annals Otology, Rhinology and Laryngology. 2012; 21(7):431-434.